Understanding
Echinacea

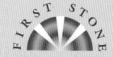

Contents

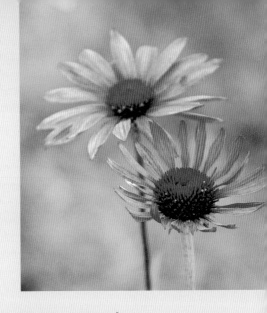

1 Introducing Echinacea

Echinacea is a born-again natural remedy that has an astonishing number of healing qualities.

Echinacea (pronounced eck-in-asia) fights viruses and fungi; it is antiseptic, anti-inflammatory and anti-oxidant. It can help to lower or raise abnormal body temperature and is even able to encourage the body to change the course of a disease.

The success of echinacea today is linked to the widespread use of antibiotics in medicine. The discovery of the power of antibiotics led to doctors being besieged by

It can encourage the body to change the course of a disease

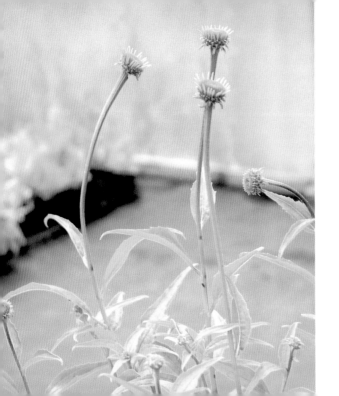

The quest is on to find an alternative to antibiotics.

patients demanding the 'magic bullet'. For decades, thinking it could do no harm, doctors prescribed antibiotics for the most trivial complaints.

We now know to our cost that this indiscriminate use of antibiotics has done a lot of harm. Mutant genes have become resistant to antibiotics, drug-resistant bacteria have sprung up, and life-threatening microbes are waging war against antibiotics that were supposed to control them.

Add to this the alarming fact that plague is no longer confined to the history books and it is hardly surprising that people feel the need to search for alternatives.

This quest has seen a rising interest in natural healing methods, with the value of herbs such as echinacea being rediscovered.

The last decade has seen soaring worldwide sales of echinacea, reflecting its reputation as a master regulator of the immune system and the king of blood purifiers.

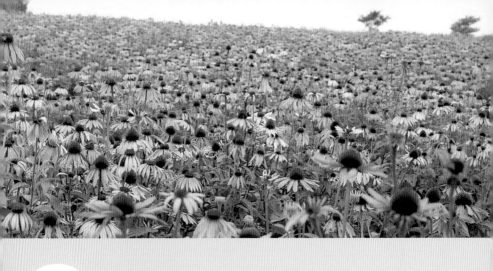

2 A Brief History

Echinacea's natural habitat is the Central Plains of North America.

It was hugely popular with the Native Americans for the simple reason that they found it to be highly effective against a wide range of afflictions.

- The Cheyenne used it for sore mouths and gums.
- The Choctaw used it for coughs and dyspepsia.
- The Comanche used it for toothache and sore throats.
- The Sioux used it for snakebite, blood poisoning and also rabies.
- The Dakota used it for bowel complaints, hydrophobia, old wounds, inflammation, tonsillitis, toothache, snakebite and 'distemper in horses'.

Indian braves used echinacea juice to protect hands, mouth and feet from hot coals and ceremonial fires.

They revered the herb so much that the witchdoctors used it as an offering to the spirit world. It was often added to strengthen other herbal concoctions. Unfortunately, much of the wisdom about the use of echinacea was killed off as the Europeans moved west across the Great Plains. The European settlers in America considered the Native Americans ignorant savages, and ridiculed their ancient wisdom as primitive and worthless.

The people of 'civilised' Europe very nearly succeeded in completely destroying the culture of a proud and wise people.

One of the few people of European descent to take an interest in the ways of the Native American Indians was Melvin Randolph Gilmore. He wrote:

> *The people of the European race in coming to the New World have not sought to make friends of the native population, or to make adequate use of the plants or the animals indigenous to this continent, but rather to exterminate everything found here and to supplant it with the plants and animals to which they were accustomed at home*

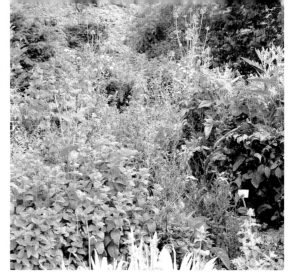

The healing power of herbs is well documented in folklore, but now scientific studies are underlining their value.

In the mid 1870s, the German physician Dr. H.C.F Meyer was introduced to echinacea by the Pawnee Indians living in Nebraska. He developed Meyer's Blood Purifier, which featured echinacea as one of its main ingredients. It was widely touted as a 'cure-all' and was exceptionally popular, possibly due to Meyer's extravagant claims. The label read:

> *Take one ounce three times every day in the following cases: rheumatism, sick headaches, dyspepsia, old sores and bites, open wounds, dizziness and scrofula. In case of poisoning, take the double dose and for bites of rattlesnakes take three ounces three times a day until the swelling is gone. This is an absolute cure within 24 hours.*

This was the original 'snake oil' remedy! Fortunately, some more serious manufacturers developed an interest in echinacea.

Amongst these were the 'Eclectic Physicians', of whom the most important were John King, author of the *American Dispensatory* (1852), and John Uri Lloyd.

The latter was one of the founders of the respected Lloyd Brothers Pharmaceutical Company of Cincinnati, Ohio. Echinacea became their top-selling product.

THE ECLECTICS

The Eclectics were formed in the latter part of the 18th century by Wooster Beach. While they had their roots in orthodox medicine, they became disenchanted with it and formed the school of 'Reformed Medicine'.

Its supporters became known as the Eclectics. They were major contributors to the development of herbal medicine, carrying out many studies on the effectiveness of herbal preparations in healing.

They were a major force in bringing echinacea to the forefront of herbal medicine. Echinacea became the most important herb of the Eclectic era.

Like many herbs, echinacea's popularity has waxed and waned over the years. Although favoured by Native Americans and herbalists, echinacea was condemned by orthodox medicine as a quack remedy. It staged a recovery in the early part of the 20th century, but was then dismissed as worthless by the

American Medical Association – and of course the discovery of penicillin swept aside many herbal remedies. Fortunately, echinacea has re-emerged to become one of the most popular herbs on the market with US sales alone totalling over $400 million.

THE SPREAD TO EUROPE

While the popularity of echinacea was in decline in America, it was on the rise in Germany. During the 1930s Dr. Gerhard Madhaus began researching and working with echinacea. He isolated a preparation called Echinacin, which was made from the juice of the flowers, leaves and stems of one of the varieties of *echinacea purpurea*.

Madhaus, a leading herbal medicine manufacturer from Cologne, originally went to America looking for the seeds of the most popular American variety of echinacea, *echinacea augustifolia*, but was mistakenly given seeds of the less popular *purpurea* variety.

Germany has continued to produce *echinacea purpurea* in

large quantities and has introduced it to a wider European market.

There have been many positive research studies carried out in Germany since 1939, mainly using the Echinacin developed by Madhaus.

In Europe, *echinacea purpurea* is widely used in pharmaceutical products such as toothpaste, creams, ointments and liquids for external application. It is also sold in ampoules for intravenous and intramuscular injections (this is only permitted in certain European countries). According to Bauer and Wagner, there were over 280 echinacea pharmaceutical products on sale in the 1990s and the figure is growing annually.

Echinacea is today the primary remedy for minor respiratory infections in Germany, where over 2.5 million prescriptions are issued annually. Research in Germany has concentrated on the ability of echinacea to boost the immune system.

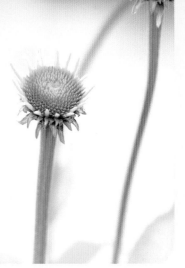

Inside
Echinacea

The name echinacea comes from the Greek name 'echinos', meaning hedgehog or sea urchin – a reference to the prickly scales of the cone-shaped seed head.

Echinacea is part of the daisy family and its bloom resembles a large daisy, with colours ranging from white to purple.

While there are nine species of echinacea, only three are commonly used as medicinal herbs:

Echinacea augustifolia is the most popular variety in use in America. It has narrow leaves and is the smallest of the three varieties, generally growing no more than 18ins (45cm) in height.

Echinacea purpurea, the most popular variety in Europe, grows considerably taller at heights of up to 5ft (1.5m). It has a shorter purple/black root and large, somewhat hairy leaves.

Echinacea pallida in theory is the least used of the medicinal echinaceas, however it is often mistakenly sold as *echinacea augustifolia*. It grows between 2-4ft (60-120cm) tall.

Common names for echinacea include Purple Coneflower, Kansas Snake Root, Black Sampson, Sampson Root, Red Sunflower, Kansas Niggerhead, Sacred Plant and Hairs of Grandmother's Head.

GROWING ECHINACEA
Echinacea has grown in the wild in the Central Plains of North America for many hundreds of years. It's a perennial plant that prefers

AMAZING ECHINACEA

Echinacea is toxic to mosquitoes. Take it regularly and the mosquitos are less likely to find you attractive enough to bite.

dry and open areas. The seeds should be spread out without being pushed into the soil. The plant thrives in full sun. Autumn is the best time to harvest if you decide to grow your own.

CHEMISTRY
From a healing point of view, the most important constituents of echinacea are:

- Caffeic acid derivatives, which are sometimes called echinacosides (these are believed to have antibiotic properties)
- Volatile oils
- Polysaccharides
- Polyines
- Polyenes
- Isobutylamides.

It is the latter that is responsible for the tingling or numbing sensation on the tongue (especially pronounced from *echinacea augustifolia*).

However, researchers Bauer and Wagner believe that it is not one substance that is responsible for the healing properties of echinacea, but a synergy that exists between the plant's many components.

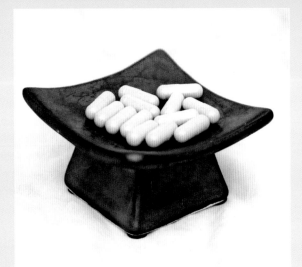

4 Boosting Immunity

Echinacea is most famous for its effect on the immune system. Let's take a look at how this system works to keep your body healthy.

It's your immune system that fights off all the bacteria, viruses, microbes, protozoa, parasites, tumours and other invaders that are intent on attacking you, or taking up residence in your body.

The immune system also cleans up dead cells and toxic waste products, and offers protection against radiation and chemical pollutants.

A healthy immune system can make 2,000 new immune cells every second. That multiplies to 120,000 every minute and 7,200,000 every hour. What commanding officer wouldn't be happy with that turnover of fresh troops?

A GUIDED TOUR OF YOUR IMMUNE ARMY

Every second of every day, your immune system is waging war on your behalf. The resulting conflicts could rival any *Star Wars* film.

21

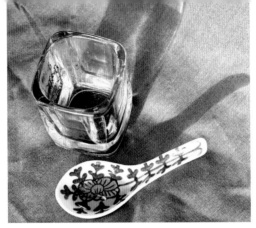

Natural healing: Echinacea, here shown in tincture form, stimulates the body's immune system.

Below are listed some of the front-line troops that make up your immune army.

THE WHITE BLOOD CELLS
(Leucocytes)

These operate where most of the fighting takes place. Your white blood cells are divided into separate fighting units:

- T-lymphocytes
- B-lymphocytes
- Macrophages
- Polymorphs.

T-lymphocytes
These are under orders from the thymus gland, the master gland of the immune system.

- Some, like the T-helper cells, are on red alert, looking out for invaders, ready to mobilise your immune system.
- Others, like the T-suppressor cells, are designed to switch off the immune system once the battle is over.
- Cytotoxic T-cells are like the SAS. They search out and destroy viruses and other invaders that have hidden inside your cells.
- Lymphokine-producing T-cells are also killer cells, but they are targeted to kill invaders that move in between the cells.

B-lymphocytes
The B-cells can either work with the other cells of the immune system or they can go freelance.

Primarily, the B-lymphocytes attach themselves to invaders, and make antibodies to render them harmless until a macrophage or polymorph comes along to gobble them up. One of the strengths of the B-lymphocytes is that they 'remember' the invader and are ready to deal with it should it try to attack you again.

This ensures that you don't usually succumb to the same bug again – for example, it's unusual to get measles twice.

③ *Macrophages*

These are the chameleons of our immune army. They can change their shape and function as required and have receptors on the surface of their cells to allow them to recognise invaders.

They are a mobile chemical factory, capable of making up to 40 different enzymes and proteins that will destroy invaders. Macrophages are incredibly house-proud. They are like the 'Pacmen' of the immune system and go around gobbling up invaders and tidying up the blood and lymph by removing any debris or chemical waste.

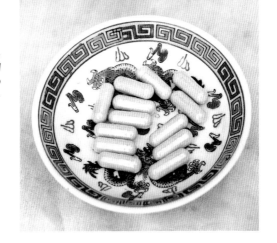

*Taking the medicine:
Some people find
capsules easier to
swallow than tablets.*

Polymorphs

Polymorphs are like robots that are programmed to destroy. Inside polymorphs are little bags of enzymes called lysosomes, which are powerful enough to kill invaders. Unfortunately the lysosomes are so powerful and the polymorphs so gung ho, that

25

they often end up on a kamikaze mission.

FLOWER POWER
You have had but a glimpse of the complex and diverse methods by which your immune system protects you from illness.

If you want to remain in good health, it is certainly in your best interest to ensure that your immune system is operating at maximum efficiency.

Diet, exercise and a healthy lifestyle are obviously key, but

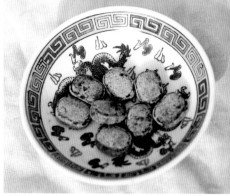

Soothing: You can even find echinacea in the form of a throat-easing lozenge.

immune-regulating herbs like echinacea can also help.

Echinacea is effective against viral and fungal infections as well as bacterial infections.

Not only does it help fight infection and kill bacteria, it also strengthens the immune system, helping it to work more efficiently.

HERE'S HOW IT WORKS

• Echinacea modulates antibody binding sites. Antibodies are sticky projections that latch on to infectious invaders and tag them. This has a dual purpose: it renders them harmless and ensures they will be recognised quickly next time.

• Echinacea's effectiveness in stopping the spread of bacteria is due in no small measure to its effect of reducing the production of hyaluronidase.

This is an enzyme which stops hyaluronic acid from gluing cells together to create healthy tissue that can't be penetrated by invaders. Unchecked, this enzyme makes cells porous and susceptible to bacterial invasion.

• Studies have shown that the

echinacoside and caffeic acid content of echinacea in particular inhibit the growth of bacteria such as *Staphylococcus aureus*, *Corneybacterium diptheria* and *Proteus vulgaris*.

- Another of echinacea's strengths as an anti-bacterial is its ability to maximise efficiency of the production of fibrinoblasts. Fibrinoblasts make collagen, which in turn forms new tissue, which will protect against invasion. Echinacea also contains the important anti-oxidant vitamins A, C and E.

- It mobilises the body's white blood cells – our immune army.

- It encourages an increase in the macrophages that go around gobbling up the enemy.

- Echinacea has been shown in laboratory tests to contain interferon-like properties. Interferon is a naturally occurring chemical which boosts immune function. Interferon is produced by the T-helper cells and is being studied for its potential in treating cancer.

- Echinacea's activation of the 'alternative complement pathway' is thought to be responsible for its antimicrobial and anti-cancer properties. A major polysaccharide component of echinacea, called inulin, activates this alternative complement pathway.

- Echinacea increases properdin levels. Properdin is a protein in human blood that is the body's natural activator of the alternative complement pathway.

- Echinacea also has a mild antibiotic effect.

ECHINACEA, THE KING OF BLOOD PURIFIERS

Battles fought by the immune system leave a lot of cellular debris and toxic waste behind, and here echinacea comes into its own. Echinacea helps to stimulate the flow of lymphatic fluids by improving filtration and drainage.

Echinacea's ability to aid in the removal of toxic waste from the blood cannot be underestimated. Undoubtedly, this is why echinacea has won the reputation as the king of blood purifiers.

Echinacea has also earned the reputation of behaving like cortisone because of its ability to stimulate the adrenal cortex. This cortisone-like action would explain some of its anti-inflammatory activity.

ECHINACEA CAN HELP FIGHT...

RESPIRATORY INFECTIONS
Respiratory infections can have bacterial, viral and/or fungal ingredients. This versatile herb has earned a reputation for its ability to treat respiratory infections including: influenza, tonsillitis, bronchitis, colds and whooping cough.

CHRONIC FATIGUE
It is my belief that chronic fatigue can result from the body's inability to deal effectively with toxins.

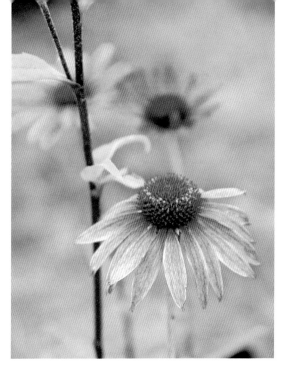

*In the pink:
Echinacea bears the
common name of
Coneflower in many
of its natural
habitats.*

Most toxins are stored in the connective tissue and when this gets clogged up information from the body's "electrical messengers" is either undeliverable or gets scrambled en route.

Echinacea's ability to clean up cellular debris and purify the blood are of obvious benefit in this condition.

ALLERGIES

Echinacea's ability to regulate the immune system makes it a useful herb for reducing the inflammatory symptoms associated with allergies.

ENLARGED PROSTATE

Echinacea's ability to reduce swelling is also thought to be due to its anti-inflammatory properties. Because of this it is believed to be one of the most powerful herbs available for use in the treatment of enlarged prostate.

CANCER

Researchers have discovered that echinacea contains a tumour-inhibiting compound.

However, while further

research may lead to the use of echinacea in cancer treatment in the future, it should *NOT* be considered a substitute for conventional medicine.

AIDS

There is conflicting evidence relating to using echinacea in the treatment of Aids.

Some say it is beneficial, while others say it lowers favourable T-cell ratios. Research continues. In the meantime, those suffering with Aids should continue to follow their doctor's treatment.

AUTOIMMUNE CONDITIONS

There are also conflicting views on the benefits of using echinacea with autoimmune conditions (rheumatoid arthritis, multiple sclerosis, lupus etc.).

First and foremost, it is important to follow your doctor's advice. Never take alternatives without proper consultation. Some experts say you shouldn't use an immune stimulant for a condition where the immune system is already overactive, whilst others say that echinacea's ability to act as an 'alterative' rules out that concern.

Many practitioners have been prescribing echinacea for autoimmune conditions for years with successful results.

ECHINACEA CAN ALSO BE EFFECTIVE AGAINST…
- Abscesses
- Acne
- Bedsores
- Boils
- Burns
- Eczema
- Fevers
- Flatulence
- Fungal infections
- Herpes simplex
- Indigestion
- Insect bites
- Open sores
- Pelvic Inflammatory Disease
- Psoriasis
- Sore throat
- Spider bites
- Swollen glands
- Tooth and or gum disease

A PRESCRIPTION
FOR A PROBLEM

While there is evidence that certain serious illnesses have responded well to treatment with echinacea, it must be stressed that it would be extremely unwise to self-diagnose, start taking echinacea and stop taking medicine prescribed by a doctor.

If you are concerned about any aspect of your health, please consult your doctor.

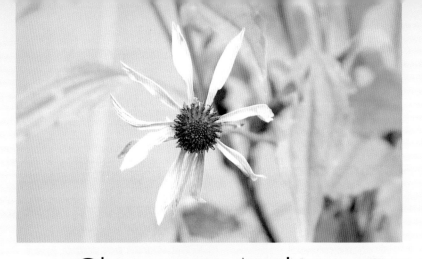

Choosing And Using Echinacea

While echinacea has powerful properties when taken internally, it can also be used externally on sores, wounds or infections.

The Native Americans used echinacea freely on snake and insect bites.

It can also be used on cuts, abscesses or boils.

If you are using echinacea externally, many experts reckon that you will get even greater benefit if you take the herb internally at the same time.

WHICH IS THE BEST ECHINACEA?

Echinacea augustifolia is the preferred variety in America and *echinacea purpurea* is the preferred variety in Europe.

There is ample evidence to prove that both are effective. *Echinacea augustifolia* is more expensive, perhaps because there is less yield per plant.

Cost aside, it really is Hobson's choice. If you asked a hundred practitioners, it would probably be close to 50:50 in favour of each of the two major varieties. One

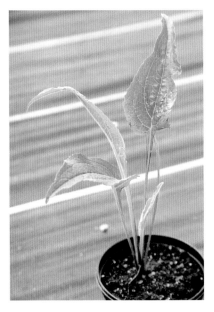

Echinacea purpurea is the preferred variety in Europe.

option is to choose a blend of the two, plus the less well-known *echinacea pallida*. There are many of these blends on the market.

Like most herbs, echinacea is available in a variety of preparations. Whatever type you choose, be it in capsule, tablet, tea, tincture, essence, bath,

AMAZING
ECHINACEA

On certain ceremonial occasions, Native Americans would often chew raw echinacea root to numb their mouths. They could put burning coals in their mouths without pain or injury. While I certainly don't recommend that you 'try this at home', you can see the potential for toothache or any other mouth pain.

compress, poultice or ointment form, the product is only as good as the quality of the raw herb from which it was made. Most practitioners insist that echinacea should be from a certified organic plant source. Good echinacea will always leave a tingling feeling on the tongue.

Echinacea tablets can be used as a means of keeping the immune system in tip-top condition.

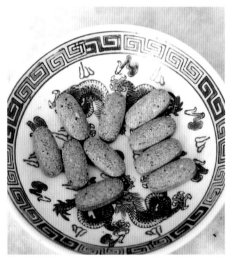

DOSAGE

Echinacea can be used in several ways and in many different forms.

As an immune system regulator, it is best to seek the advice and guidance of a qualified practitioner, as dosages vary according to the product and the brand. This particularly applies when giving echinacea to children.

Although there are conflicting opinions on how long echinacea can safely be taken for, current research indicates that there are no problems associated with long-term use, as was believed previously.

TINCTURE OF ECHINACEA
As a preventive, drops of tincture in water work well, and can be taken throughout the cold and flu season.

If you have caught an infection of any kind, echinacea can also be taken several times daily.

In both cases, it is advised that you consult your practitioner for dosage advice.

OTHER PREPARATIONS
Echinacea is also popular in capsule or tablet form. As a rough guide, 2 capsules or 1 tablet are approximately equivalent to 1 dropperful of tincture. However, this varies

41

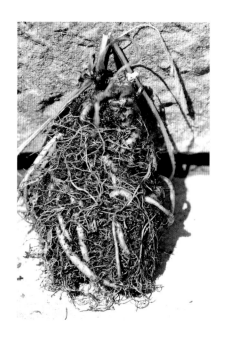

Wonder root: You can prepare the natural root of echinacea (left) or take a short cut with capsules (right).

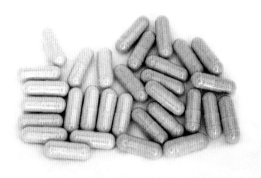

Echinacea root capsules (left) or echinacea root and leaf (right).

according to brand, so always consult your practioner.

To make your own extract of echinacea root, put 2 teaspoons in 1 cup of water and slowly bring to the boil. Allow to simmer for 10-15 minutes. This can be taken 3 times a day.

SAFETY

Echinacea is non-toxic. It can be safely used in high doses during acute infections when taken orally.

However, studies in

Germany using injectable preparations of echinacea have observed a number of side effects.

These include shivering, fever and muscle weakness, and are thought to be associated with the migration of activated T-helper cells to targeted organs.

Extremely high oral doses have occasionally caused nausea, increased urination, and dizziness, but no poisoning has been noted, even in high doses.

According to the American Botanical Council, "studies indicate little need for concern regarding the safety of echinacea".

This does not include anyone who suffers from a kidney or liver disorder, who should always consult their doctor before using echinacea or any other alternative medication.

In all cases, it is advisable to consult with a qualified practitioner if you are in any doubt about any aspect of your health, or the dosage required in a specific situation.

USEFUL COMBINATIONS

Echinacea with…

CHICKWEED
When combined with chickweed, echinacea has been used to promote weight loss.

BURDOCK ROOT
This combination is useful for treating skin eruptions.

GOLDENSEAL
Many cold remedies combine echinacea with goldenseal: goldenseal's more powerful antibiotic properties complement the more immune-stimulating properties of echinacea.

This type of preparation is especially beneficial once someone is in the throes of an infection.

CLEAVERS, POKE ROOT, WILD INDIGO and YELLOW DOCK
Use 1 part of each to 2 parts of echinacea. Make into a tea and drink 3 times daily to counteract ringworm or other fungal infections.

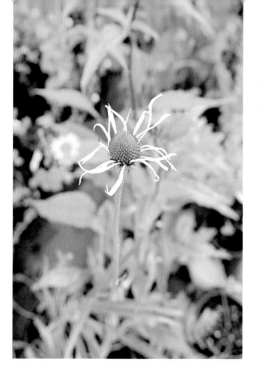

Partners in wellness: Echinacea can be combined with other herbal ingredients to make effective natural remedies.

MARIGOLD AND MYRRH
Used in equal parts with echinacea and applied externally as a lotion or tincture to ringworm or other fungal infections.

COMFREY
Mix 1 tablespoon of extract with 1 tablespoon of echinacea root extract.

Add just enough boiling water to make a paste. Allow to steep for 10 minutes.

This is an excellent treatment for cleaning and healing wounds.

Apply directly to the affected area. Cover with gauze or a bandage and leave in place for at least 30 mins.

KITCHEN HERBS
We shouldn't overlook kitchen herbs such as ginger, garlic and cayenne in combination with echinacea when fighting an infection.

POWDERED COSMETIC CLAY
When mixed with echinacea tincture, this makes an excellent poultice for boils, acne, insect bites or stings.

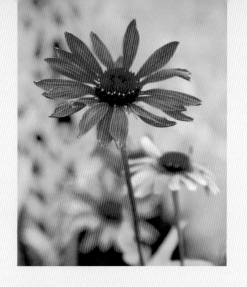

6 What They Say About Echinacea

While historical and anecdotal evidence highlight the wide-ranging uses of echinacea, scientific studies in the last 10 years have tended to focus on the immune-boosting properties of the plant.

In 1992, Braunig and others carried out a double-blind, placebo-controlled trial involving 180 volunteers to study the effects of an *echinacea purpurea* root alcohol extract in relieving the symptoms and duration of flu-like symptoms. In double-blind, placebo-controlled trials, in order to ensure consistency, no one knows who is receiving what until the end of the trial.

When the trial was completed, it was discovered that the volunteers who had been receiving 900mg/dose (equivalent to roughly 4 droppersful) showed a statistically significant improvement compared to the placebo group.

However, volunteers who received only half that dose (450mg/dose) showed improvements that were only comparable to those in the placebo group. This study highlights the importance of getting the dosage right if you expect echinacea to have an immune-boosting effect.

SUSCEPTIBILITY

Another study examined volunteers who were deemed to have a greater susceptibility to infections (determined by a low T4/T8 cell ratio in the blood).

In all, 108 patients were studied and divided into two groups: group A 'control' and group B 'treatment'. They received a dose of between 2-4ml/day of either echinacea or placebo.

The treatment (echinacea) group showed significant results: a decrease in the frequency of infections, a reduction in the average duration of colds, and less severe symptoms.

The placebo group showed no significant results.

TESTIMONIALS

A practitioner called Dr.

Ellingwood, who died in 1920, recorded the treatment of a 45-year-old man who was suffering from the after-effects of being vaccinated with a supposed impure virus.

He began to exhibit unusual symptoms and his vitality began to wane.

His hair came out, his nails began to fall off, and he developed skin problems and eye problems for which he was referred to Professor Martin, President of the Chicago Ophthalmic College.

Professor Martin prescribed 10 grains of iodide of potassium daily and fed him freely on phospho-albumin.

The loss of hair stopped, but no other favourable results were noted.

Professor Martin called in Dr. Ellingwood.

The prognosis for the patient did not look good, but as a last resort, Dr. Ellingwood suggested using echinacea at the dose of 20 drops every 4 hours and the phospho-albumin alone to be continued.

Within 4 weeks, not only

had the patient regained his normal body weight but his other symptoms had also disappeared.

Dr. Ellingwood also had this to say about echinacea:

"For 20 to 25 years, echinacea has been passing through the stages of critical experimentation under the observation of several thousand physicians, and its remarkable properties are receiving positive confirmation.

"As yet, but few disparaging statements have been made.

"All who use it correctly fall quickly into line as enthusiasts in its praise.

"The experience of the writer is similar to that of the rest."

Modern-day practitioners are also convinced by echinacea.

Andrea Watson, a medical herbalist from Canada, says:

"I have been using and prescribing echinacea for over 15 years.

"It is one of the most versatile and powerful herbs I use in my clinic.

"I recommend echinacea for resistance to infection and many other serious illnesses.

"It is also a very good purifier of the blood and the lymphatic system.

"Every time I prescribe echinacea, I am confident of a good result".

I practise both conventional and alternative medicine. The use of herbs is a very important and effective part of my treatment protocol. Echinacea is amongst the most useful and versatile of all the herbs I use. One of the most impressive features of echinacea is its ability to build up the body's natural resistance to germs and infection

Dr. David Armitage
British doctor and medical herbalist

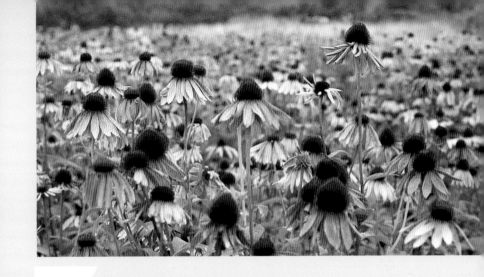

7 Conservation

Echinacea's enormous popularity, combined with the fact that it grows naturally in the wild, has led to the herb becoming endangered.

A Native American described echinacea digging on her reservation as having all the hallmarks of the gold rush mentality: "They drive through fences, dig holes, don't cover them and drive off with car trunks full of the stuff".

Echinacea in the wild has all but disappeared in many areas. The problem has become so bad that some varieties have been awarded endangered species status in some US states.

INITIATIVES
Conservation initiatives have included a donation from employees of American Airlines, who contributed $200,000 towards the purchase of the 43-acre Couchville cedar glade, home to one of the largest enclaves of wild echinacea.

The money was collected through a can recycling

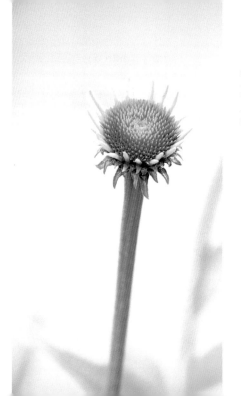

Under threat: Echinacea growing wild in its native habitat is coming under threat from unscrupulous people in search of a free "harvest" of this popular herb.

programme run on the airlines' planes.

COMMERCIAL CULTIVATION

With popularity for echinacea growing annually, the only way to meet demand and protect the existing species in the wild would seem to be to encourage commercial cultivation.

Many tobacco growers have been scared by the huge payouts to lung cancer victims, and US government initiatives include encouraging farmers to grow echinacea as an alternative crop to tobacco.

Hopefully a solution will be found, so that we can benefit from the powers of this truly amazing herb without having to worry about its future.

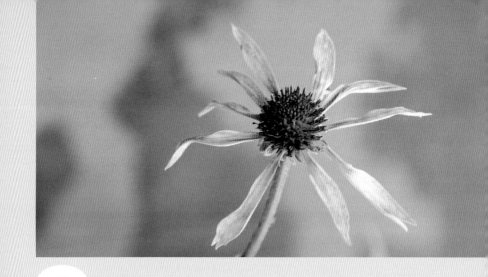

8 Resources

FURTHER READING

Indian Medicine For The Immune System
Dr. Desmond Corrigan
Amberwood Publishing
ISBN 0951772376

Echinacea – The Plant That Boosts Your Immune System
Douglas Schar
Souvenir Press
ISBN 0285634887

Echinacea, The Immune Herb
Christopher Hobbs
Botanica Press
ISBN 1884360033

Echinacea, Nature's Immune Enhancer
Steven Foster
Inner Tradition International
ISBN 0892813865

Your Complete Guide to Echinacea and Immunity (Natural Pharmacist Guide)
Elizabeth Collins, Nancy Berkoff
Random House
ISBN 0761515585

User's Guide to Echinacea and Other Cold and Flu Fighters
Laurel Vukovic
Basic Health Publications
ISBN 1591200849

Herbs for Health: A Handy Pocket Guide for Knowing and Using 50 Common Herbs
Steven Foster
Interweave Press
ISBN 1883010276

WEBSITES

American Botantical Council
www.herbalgram.org

A non-profit education and research organisation, which aims to be a prime source of information on the safe and effective use of medicinal plants.

The ABC's mission is to educate the public so that ordinary people can make responsible choices about herbal medicine as an accepted part of healthcare.

Herb Research Foundation
www.herbs.org
A source of science-based information on the health benefits and safety aspects of herbs.

The HRF produces Health Information Packets on herbs, specific health conditions and related topics. These are deliverable by e-mail.

AMAZING ECHINACEA

Echinacea was often used in witchcraft to strengthen the power of spells. Native American witchdoctors used it as a precious offering to the spirit world.

About the author

Marjorie Green is a practitioner, writer and lecturer on Clinical Nutrition, Bioenergetic Medicine, Neuro Linguistic Programming and Emotional Freedom Techniques. She has made many appearances on television and radio.

She can be contacted via e-mail: marjoriecgreen@aol.com

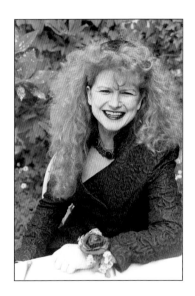

Other titles in the series

- Understanding Acupressure
- Understanding Acupuncture
- Understanding The Alexander Technique
- Understanding Aromatherapy
- Understanding Bach Flower Remedies
- Understanding Evening Primrose
- Understanding Feng Shui
- Understanding Fish Oils
- Understanding Garlic
- Understanding Ginseng
- Understanding Head Massage
- Understanding Kinesiology
- Understanding Lavender
- Understanding Massage
- Understanding Pilates
- Understanding Reflexology
- Understanding Reiki
- Understanding St. John's Wort
- Understanding Shiatsu
- Understanding Yoga

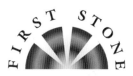

First published in 2004 by First Stone Publishing
PO Box 8, Lydney, Gloucestershire, GL15 6YD United Kingdom

The contents of this book are for information only and are not intended as a substitute for appropriate medical attention. The author and publishers admit no liability for any consequences arising from following any advice contained within this book. If you have any concerns about your health or medication, always consult your doctor.

ISBN 1 904439 18 7

Printed and bound in Hong Kong through Printworks International Ltd.